EFFORTLESS WEIGHT LOSS

A Step-by-Step Guide to a Healthier lifestyle

Mariee Sunny

Copyright © 2023 by Mariee Sunny

This book is for informational purposes only and does not constitute medical or professional advice. The author and publisher make no representations or warranties with respect to the accuracy or completeness of the contents of this book and specifically disclaim any implied warranties of merchantability or fitness for any particular purpose. The author and publisher shall not be liable for any loss of profit or any other commercial damages, including but not limited to special, incidental, consequential, or other damages.

ACKNOWLEDGMENTS:

I am incredibly grateful to the many people who have supported me throughout the writing of this weight loss book.

First and foremost, I would like to thank all of the individuals who have struggled with their weight and shared their experiences with me. Your courage and honesty have been a constant source of inspiration and motivation for me, and I am honored to have been able to share your stories and insights with others.

I am deeply grateful to my editor, whose invaluable guidance and feedback helped to shape and refine this book into its final form. Your wisdom, patience, and expertise have been truly invaluable, and I am proud to have worked with you.

I also want to extend my heartfelt appreciation to the many researchers, scientists, and health professionals who have dedicated their lives to understanding the complex relationship between diet, exercise, and weight loss. Your tireless work has been instrumental in shaping the knowledge and recommendations presented in this book, and I am honored to have been able to draw upon your expertise.

Finally, I would like to thank my family and friends for their unwavering love and support throughout this journey. Your belief in me and my work has meant the world to me, and I could not have done this without you.

To everyone who has contributed in some way to the creation of this weight loss book, thank you from the bottom of my heart.

Your contributions have made a difference, and I hope that this book will help others on their own journeys towards health and wellness.

TABLE OF CONTENT

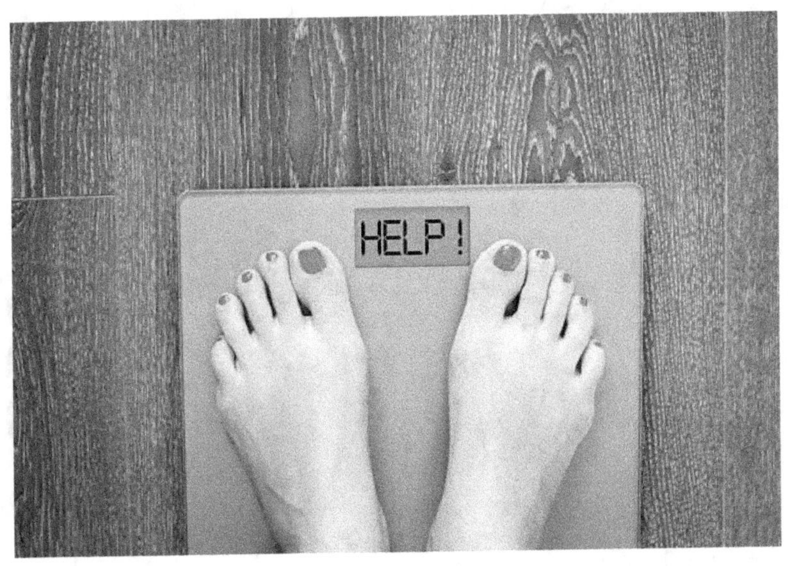
HELP !

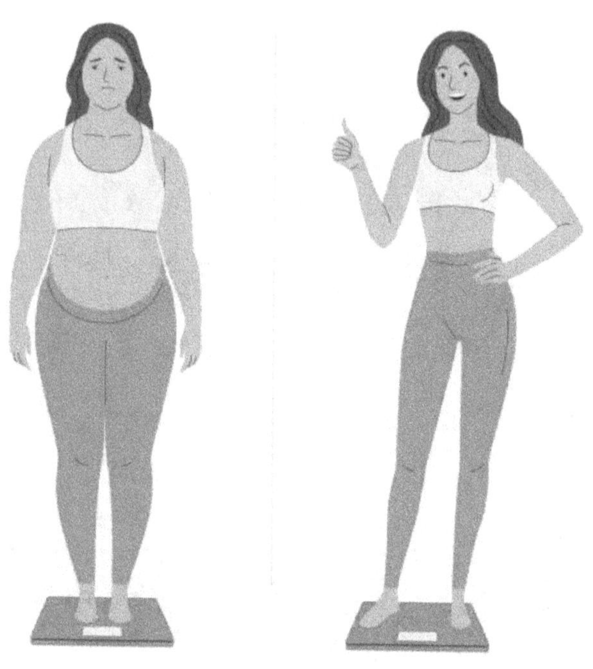

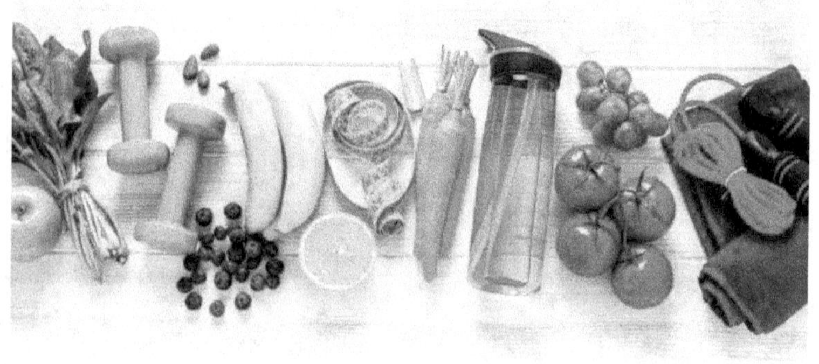

OVERVIEW:

This comprehensive non-fiction book provides a scientific approach to weight loss, addressing the most common misconceptions and providing practical tips and strategies for successful weight management.

The book covers a range of topics, from understanding the biology of weight gain and loss, to the importance of nutrition, physical activity, and behavioral change. The author provides a detailed analysis of various diets and exercise programs, and discusses the latest research on the role of genetics, hormones, and the gut micro biome in weight regulation.

Purpose:

The purpose of this book is to educate and empower readers to make informed decisions about their weight management journey. It aims to bust the myths surrounding weight loss and to provide a practical, science-based approach to losing weight and keeping it off for good. The book is suitable for people of all ages, body types, and fitness levels, and is designed to be a valuable resource for anyone looking to achieve and maintain a healthy weight. Whether you're a beginner or an experienced dieter, you'll find valuable information and practical advice to help you reach your goals. The ultimate goal of the book is to help readers achieve long-term success in their weight loss journey and to live a healthy, fulfilling life.

Understanding the Importance of Weight Loss

Weight loss is an important aspect of leading a healthy lifestyle, as excessive weight can lead to a range of health problems. Some of the reasons why weight loss is important include:

Reducing the risk of chronic diseases: Excessive weight is a major risk factor for several chronic diseases, such as Type 2 diabetes, heart disease, and some forms of cancer. By losing weight, you can lower your risk of developing these conditions.

Improving physical health: Being overweight can cause physical problems, such as joint pain, back pain, and sleep apnea. By losing weight, you can improve your physical health and reduce the chances of developing these problems.

Boosting self-esteem and confidence: Losing weight can help improve your body image and self-esteem, which can have a positive impact on your overall quality of life.

Enhancing mental health: Obesity is linked to depression and anxiety, and losing weight can help improve your mental health and wellbeing.

Living a longer life: Excessive weight is associated with a range of health problems that can shorten your lifespan. By losing weight, you can increase your chances of living a longer and healthier life.

It's important to remember that weight loss should be approached in a healthy and sustainable way, through a combination of diet and exercise. Consulting a healthcare professional can also help ensure that you are taking the right steps towards a healthier weight.

Setting Realistic Goals for Weight Loss

Here are some realistic goals suggested for you:

1.   To begin, choose a weight-loss objective that is both feasible and practical. For example, aim to lose 1-2 pounds per week for a total of 10-20 pounds in 10-20 weeks.

2.   Incorporate exercise into your daily routine, aim to achieve 30 minutes of physical activity daily, 5-6 days a week.

3.   Create a healthy meal plan that consists of nutritious foods and reduces caloric intake. Aim to have at least 5 servings of fruits and vegetables per day and limit processed foods, sugary drinks, and high-fat foods.

4.   Keep track of your food intake and monitor your weight regularly.

5.   Keep hydrate by consuming at least 8 glasses of water daily.

6.   Get enough sleep and aim to have 7-8 hours of sleep per night.

7.   Avoid skipping meals and stick to a consistent eating schedule.

8.   Seek support from friends, family, or a support group to help keep you motivated.

9.   Practice mindfulness and stress-management techniques, such as meditation or yoga, to reduce stress and maintain a healthy mindset.

10.   Celebrate small victories along the way and be kind to yourself when setbacks occur. Keep in mind that losing weight is a process rather than a final goal.

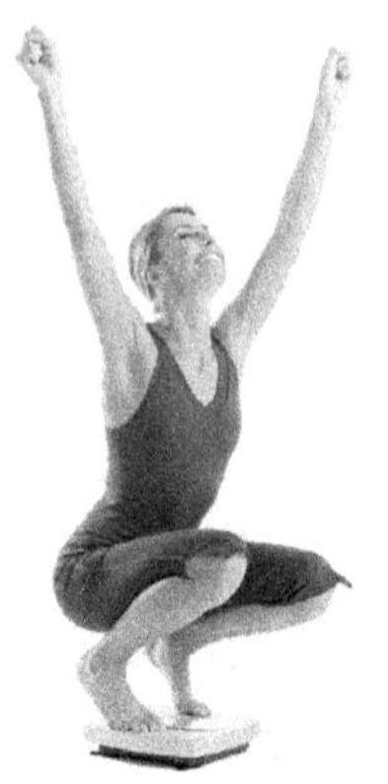

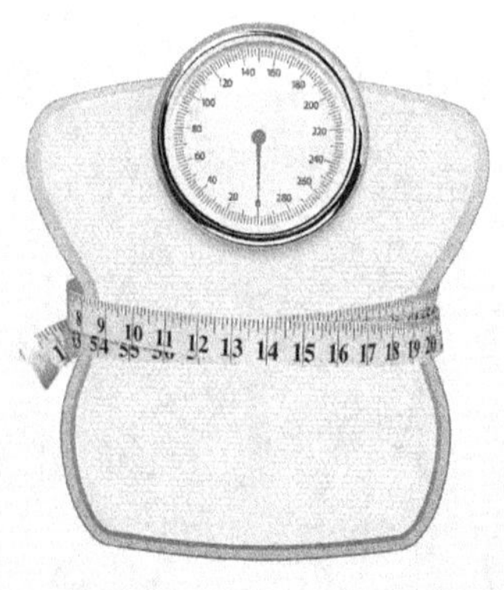

CHAPTER 1: UNDERSTANDING THE SCIENCE OF WEIGHT LOSS

How the body gains and losses weight

Weight gain and loss in the human body is a complex process that is influenced by several factors such as genetics, diet, physical activity, hormone levels, and emotional status.

When the body consumes more calories than it expends, weight gain results. The excess calories are then stored as fat, which increases the overall body weight. There are various reasons for overeating such as emotional eating, unhealthy food choices, lack of physical activity, and sedentary lifestyle.

On the other hand, weight loss occurs when the body burns more calories than it takes in. This can be accomplished by combining a nutritious diet with frequent exercise.

A diet that is rich in whole foods, lean protein, and vegetables and low in sugar and processed foods can help to reduce calorie intake and support weight loss. Regular exercise, especially strength training and cardiovascular activity, can help to increase the number of calories burned and promote weight loss.

Hormonal imbalances can also play a role in weight gain and loss. For example, changes in cortical levels, which is a stress hormone, can lead to weight gain. Thyroid dysfunction can also impact weight, as it regulates metabolism and the body's ability to burn calories.

In conclusion, weight gain and loss is a complex process that is influenced by a combination of factors such as diet, physical activity, hormone levels, and emotional status. To achieve a healthy weight, it is essential to maintain a balanced diet and engage in regular physical activity.

It is also important to seek medical advice if there is a concern about hormonal imbalances or other health issues that may impact weight.

Factors affecting weight gain and loss

Weight gain and loss are greatly influenced by various factors such as genetics, metabolism, physical activity, diet, hormonal imbalances, stress, sleep, and medications.

It is crucial to understand and address these factors to maintain a healthy weight. In same view, explained factors are:

Energy balance: This is the balance between the amount of energy taken in through food and drinks, and the amount of energy expended through physical activity and metabolic processes. A positive energy balance leads to weight gain, and a negative energy balance results in weight loss.

Genetics: Genetics play a significant role in determining an individual's body weight, body composition, and metabolism. Some people may be more susceptible to weight gain or obesity due to inherited genetic traits.

Metabolism: The rate of metabolism, or the rate at which the body burns energy, can affect weight.

People with a slower metabolism may have a harder time losing weight, as they burn fewer calories than people with a faster metabolism.

Physical activity: Physical activity plays a crucial role in weight control, as it helps to increase energy expenditure and burn more calories.

Regular exercise and physical activity can help to maintain a healthy weight or prevent weight gain.

Diet: What you eat plays a significant role in determining weight gain or loss. A diet high in calories and low in fiber, whole grains, and protein can lead to weight gain. On the other hand, a diet rich in fiber, whole grains, and protein can help with weight loss.

Sleep: Sleep plays a crucial role in regulating hormones that affect weight, such as cortisol and leptin. Lack of sleep can cause an increase in cortisol levels, leading to weight gain, while adequate sleep can help regulate hormones and promote weight loss.

Hormonal imbalances: Hormonal imbalances, such as those associated with hypothyroidism, polycystic ovary syndrome (PCOS), and menopause, can cause weight gain or difficulty losing weight.

Medications: Certain medications, such as steroids and antidepressants, can cause weight gain. It is important to discuss the potential side effects of any medications with your healthcare provider.

Stress: Chronic stress can cause an increase in cortisol levels, leading to weight gain. Stress also can trigger overeating, which can contribute to weight gain.

Age: As people age, their metabolism naturally slows down, making it harder to maintain a healthy weight. Additionally, muscle mass decreases with age, which can further slow down metabolism and contribute to weight gain.

The Role of Metabolism and Hormones in Weight Management

Hormones play a crucial role in regulating metabolism and weight management.

Metabolism refers to the processes by which the body converts food into energy and regulates the storage and use of that energy. Hormones are chemical messengers produced by the endocrine glands that regulate various bodily functions, including metabolism.

Here are some hormones that play a role in weight management:

Leptin: This hormone is produced by fat cells and regulates the feeling of satiety, or fullness, in the brain. Leptin signals the brain that the body has enough energy stored in fat cells, and reduces hunger and food cravings. Low levels of leptin are associated with obesity and can make it difficult to lose weight.

Ghrelin: This hormone, also known as the "hunger hormone," is produced by the stomach and stimulates hunger. Before a meal, ghrelin levels rise, and thereafter, they fall. Ghrelin levels are also linked to obesity and can make weight loss difficult by increasing hunger and food cravings.

Insulin: The pancreas secretes the hormone insulin, which controls blood sugar level. When we eat, insulin helps to transport glucose from the bloodstream into the cells for energy.

High insulin levels, especially if they persist over time, can lead to insulin resistance and contribute to weight gain.

Thyroid: Hormones produced by the thyroid gland controls the body's metabolism. Hypothyroidism, a condition in which the thyroid gland does not produce enough hormones, can lead to slow metabolism and weight gain.

In conclusion, hormones play a crucial role in regulating metabolism and weight management. Hormones such as leptin, ghrelin, insulin, and thyroid hormones are just a few examples of how hormones can affect appetite, energy expenditure, and the storage and utilization of energy in the body.

It's important to maintain a healthy balance of hormones for optimal weight management and overall health.

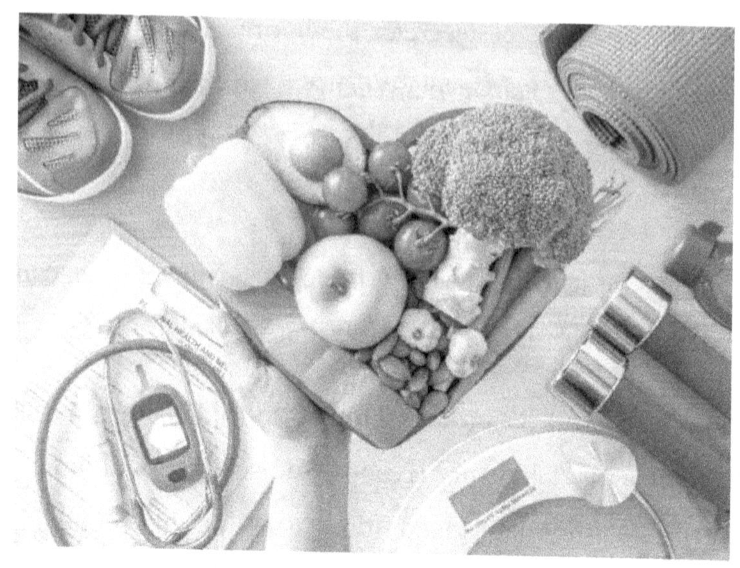

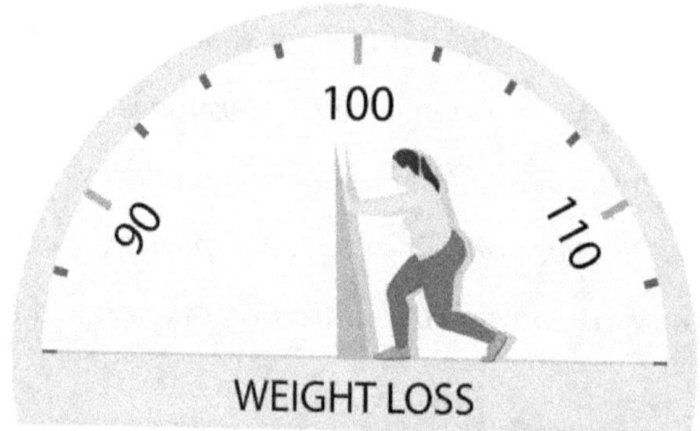

100
90
110
WEIGHT LOSS

CHAPTER 2: DEVELOPING A HEALTHY MINDSET

Overcoming emotional eating and negative self-talk

Emotional eating and negative self-talk can be two significant obstacles to a healthy lifestyle. However, with the right strategies and mindset, it's possible to overcome them and establish healthier habits. To get you started, consider the following advice:

Identify the triggers: Before you can overcome emotional eating and negative self-talk, you need to identify what triggers them. Keep a journal to track your emotions, thoughts, and food choices throughout the day. This can help you understand the patterns that lead to unhealthy habits.

Practice Mindfulness: Mindfulness is a powerful tool for managing emotions and reducing stress. When you find yourself reaching for food in response to negative thoughts or emotions, take a moment to pause and focus on your breathing. This will help you to slow down and be more mindful of your choices.

Replace negative self-talk with positive affirmations: Negative self-talk can be harmful to your self-esteem and contribute to emotional eating. Try to shift yours attention from your perceived flaws to something more positive. Write down positive affirmations that resonate with you and repeat them to yourself when you notice negative self-talk creeping in.

Find alternative coping mechanisms: Emotional eating is often a way to cope with negative emotions, but it's not a healthy solution. Instead, try to find alternative ways to manage stress, such as exercise, meditation, or talking to a friend.

Seek professional help: If you're struggling with emotional eating and negative self-talk, it's okay to seek professional help. A therapist or counselor can provide you with the support and guidance you need to make lasting changes.

In conclusion, overcoming emotional eating and negative self-talk is a journey that requires patience, perseverance, and self-compassion.

By identifying triggers, practicing mindfulness, and finding alternative coping mechanisms, you can develop healthier habits and boost your confidence and self-esteem.

Building a Positive Body Image

Building a positive body image is an important aspect of one's overall well-being and self-esteem. A positive body image is when a person views their body in a positive and accepting light, regardless of its shape, size, or perceived flaws. Some ways to help build a positive body image:

Focus on health, not appearance: Rather than focusing on your appearance, concentrate on your physical and mental health. Set achievable goals for yourself, like eating a healthy diet, getting enough sleep, and exercising regularly.

Surround yourself with positive influences: Surround yourself with people who support and encourage you, and limit exposure to negative media that may cause you to feel self-conscious or critical of your body.

Practice self-care: Take care of yourself by engaging in activities that make you feel good.

This can include things like getting a massage, taking a relaxing bath, or engaging in a hobby you enjoy.

Challenge negative self-talk: Notice and challenge any negative thoughts you have about your body. Replace these thoughts with positive affirmations and focus on your strengths and accomplishments.

Embrace your uniqueness: Embrace your individuality and all that makes you unique, including your body shape and size. Celebrate your body for all that it can do, such as running, dancing, or simply breathing.

Celebrate diversity: Recognize and celebrate the diverse shapes, sizes, and abilities of bodies in the world. This will help to challenge beauty standards and promote a more inclusive and positive view of bodies.

Remember, building a positive body image takes time and effort, but with persistence and self-compassion, it is possible. By focusing on health, positivity, and self-care, you can learn to love and appreciate your body just the way it is.

Staying Motivated and Accountable

Set realistic and measurable goals: Decide on the amount of weight you want to lose and set a deadline for achieving it. Write it down and review it regularly.

Track your progress: Use a food diary or app to record what you eat and your physical activity. Seeing your progress in black and white can be a powerful motivator.

Find a workout buddy: Having someone to exercise with can make it more fun and keep you accountable.

Reward yourself: Set up a system of rewards for reaching milestones in your weight loss journey. This could be a special treat or a new piece of clothing.

Stay positive: Stay positive and focus on what you are achieving, rather than what you are giving up.

Eat healthy: Choose nutritious, low-calorie foods and limit your portion sizes.

Stay active: Try to be physically active for at least 30 minutes a day, even if it's just a brisk walk.

Avoid temptations: Avoid tempting situations that make you want to snack or overeat.

Get enough sleep: A good night's sleep helps you maintain a healthy weight.

Surround yourself with support: Surround yourself with supportive friends and family who encourage you to stick to your weight loss goals.

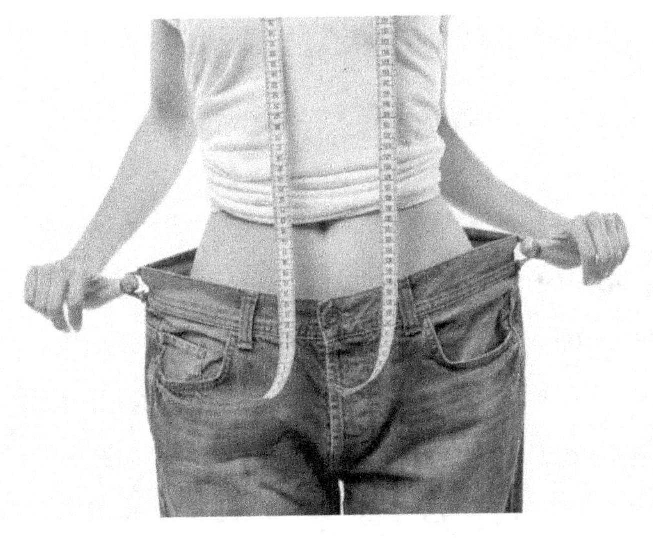

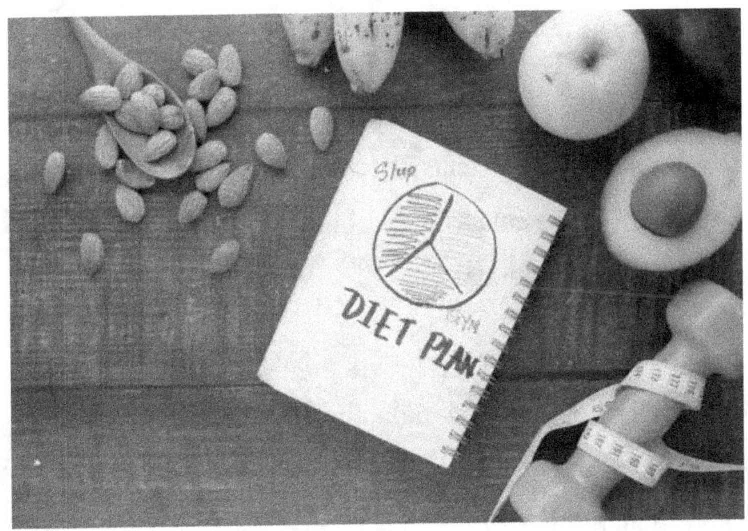
Sleep
DIET PLAN

CHAPTER 3: NUTRITIONAL STRATEGIES FOR WEIGHT LOSS

The Importance of a Balanced Diet

Balanced diet refers to a dietary pattern that includes all the essential nutrients, vitamins, and minerals in the required amounts to maintain a healthy body. In today's fast-paced world, most people tend to rely on junk food and neglect healthy eating habits. This often leads to an unhealthy lifestyle and various health issues.

Reasons why a balanced diet is so important:

Provides Essential Nutrients - A balanced diet provides all the essential nutrients that the body needs to function properly. These include carbohydrates, proteins, fats, vitamins, and minerals.

Boosts Energy Levels - Eating a balanced diet filled with essential nutrients helps to maintain a stable level of energy throughout the day, thus improving overall performance and productivity.

Supports Weight Management - A balanced diet is crucial in maintaining a healthy weight. Eating the right balance of macronutrients and limiting calorie-dense foods can help to control weight and prevent obesity.

Prevents Chronic Diseases - A diet high in saturated fats and processed foods can increase the risk of chronic diseases such as heart disease, stroke, and type 2 diabetes. A balanced diet, on the other hand, can help to reduce this risk.

Maintains Mental Health - A balanced diet can also help to maintain mental health by providing the necessary nutrients to support brain function and improve mood.

Supports Physical Health - A balanced diet plays a vital role in maintaining physical health. It can help to strengthen the immune system, improve bone health, and reduce the risk of various health conditions such as cancer, osteoporosis, and anemia.

In conclusion, a balanced diet is crucial for a healthy body and mind. It is important to make sure that you include a variety of foods from all food groups and limit processed and junk food. By doing this, you can enjoy a healthy and active lifestyle.

Understanding Macronutrients and Micronutrients

When it comes to maintaining a healthy diet, it's important to understand the role of both macro and micro nutrients. These nutrients play a vital role in supporting our overall health and well-being, and it's important to get the right balance of each to ensure we are fueling our bodies with the right nutrients.

Macro Nutrients

Macro nutrients are the three major components of our diets that provide us with energy: carbohydrates, proteins, and fats. Each of these macro nutrients serves a different purpose in the body and it's important to have a good balance of all three for optimal health.

Carbohydrates: Carbohydrates are an important source of energy for our bodies. They are found in foods such as bread, pasta, rice, fruits, and vegetables.

The body uses carbohydrates for energy, and any unused carbohydrates are stored as glycogen in the liver and muscles for later use.

Proteins: Proteins are essential for building and repairing muscle tissue. They are also involved in the production of hormones, enzymes, and other molecules. Proteins are found in foods such as meat, poultry, fish, dairy, beans, and lentils.

Fats: Fats are essential for the absorption of fat-soluble vitamins, as well as for providing the body with energy. They also play a role in hormone production and cell function. Fats are found in foods such as oils, butter, nuts, and avocados.

Micro Nutrients

Micro nutrients, on the other hand, are essential vitamins and minerals that the body needs in smaller amounts, but are still important for overall health. Examples of micro nutrients include vitamins A, C, D, E, and K, as well as minerals such as iron, calcium, and magnesium.

Vitamins: Vitamins are essential for a wide range of functions in the body, including maintaining healthy skin, vision, and bones. They also play a role in regulating metabolism, hormone production, and immune function.

Minerals: Minerals are important for a variety of functions in the body, including maintaining strong bones, regulating fluid balance, and supporting nerve and muscle function.

In conclusion, macro and micro nutrients play a vital role in maintaining overall health and wellness. To ensure you are getting the right balance of these nutrients, it's important to eat a varied and balanced diet that includes a wide range of foods. This can help ensure that you are getting all the essential nutrients you need for optimal health.

Meal Planning and Preparation

Meal planning is a simple yet effective strategy for maintaining a healthy and balanced diet. It involves taking the time to plan and prepare your meals in advance, allowing you to make healthier choices and save time and money in the long run.

Here are some key steps to get started with meal planning:

Assess your dietary needs: Consider your individual nutritional needs, food preferences, and any dietary restrictions or allergies. This will help you create a balanced meal plan that meets your specific needs.

Make a grocery list: Plan out the meals and snacks you want to prepare for the week and make a grocery list of the ingredients you'll need. This will help you save time and avoid impulse purchases at the grocery store.

Cook in bulk: Cook a large batch of food on the weekends or during your free time and divide it into individual portions for the week. This will save time and ensure you have healthy and convenient meals on hand.

Be imaginative, and don't be afraid to experiment with new ingredients and recipes: Meal planning is a great opportunity to experiment with new foods and flavors.

Stay flexible: It is okay if your meal plan changes. Life happens and sometimes plans change.

The important thing is to have a plan in place, so you can make healthier choices, even when things don't go as planned.

Meal planning is a valuable tool for anyone looking to maintain a healthy and balanced diet. Planning and preparing your meals ahead of time can guarantee that you are providing your body with the nutrition it needs to function at its peak.

Preparations and Guidelines for a Seven-day Food Plan for Weight loss:

Day 1:

Breakfast: Avocado Toast

Toast 2 slices of whole grain bread

Mash half of an avocado and spread it on top of the toast

Sprinkle with salt, pepper, and lemon juice to taste

Lunch: Grilled Chicken Salad

Grill 4 ounces of chicken breast

Serve on a bed of mixed greens with cherry tomatoes, cucumber, and red onion

Dress with a mixture of olive oil and balsamic vinegar

Dinner: Baked Salmon with Asparagus

Preheat oven to 400°F

Place 4 ounces of salmon fillet in a baking dish and top with lemon slices

Bake for 12-15 minutes or until the salmon is cooked through

Serve with a side of roasted asparagus and a quinoa salad

Day 2:

Breakfast: Yogurt Parfait

Layer Greek yogurt, mixed berries, and a handful of granola in a bowl or parfait glass

Repeat layers until ingredients are used up

Lunch: Veggie and Hummus Wrap

Spread hummus on a whole grain tortilla

Top with roasted red pepper, grilled zucchini, and red onion

To get bite-sized pieces, slice the tortilla after rolling it.

Dinner: Spaghetti Squash with Tomato Sauce

Preheat oven to 400°F

Cut a spaghetti squash in half, remove the seeds, and bake for 30-40 minutes

While the squash is cooking, prepare a simple tomato sauce by simmering canned tomatoes, garlic, and basil

Use a fork to scrape out the spaghetti squash and serve with the tomato sauce

Day 3:

Breakfast: Smoothie Bowl

Blend frozen mixed berries, Greek yogurt, almond milk, and a scoop of protein powder in a blender

Pour into a bowl and top with granola and sliced banana

Lunch: Turkey and Veggie Stir Fry

Cook 4 ounces of sliced turkey breast in a wok or large pan

Add a mixture of vegetables, such as broccoli, bell peppers, and onion, and stir fry for 2-3 minutes

Serve over brown rice

Dinner: Stuffed Bell Peppers

Preheat oven to 375°F

Remove the tops and seeds from 4 bell peppers.

Fill each pepper with a mixture of cooked ground turkey, brown rice, and tomato sauce

Place the peppers in a baking dish and bake for 25-30 minutes.

Day 4:

Breakfast: Oatmeal with Nuts and Berries

Cook oats according to package instructions

Stir in a handful of mixed nuts and berries before serving

Lunch: Lentil Soup

Cook lentils, carrots, celery, and onion in a large pot

Season with spices, such as thyme and rosemary, and simmer for 30 minutes

Enjoy with crusty whole grain bread

Dinner: Grilled Pork Chops with Roasted Sweet Potato

Grill 4 ounces of pork chops

Roast a sweet potato in the oven or on the grill until tender

Green beans, steamed, should be served alongside.

Day 5:

Breakfast: Egg and Vegetable Scramble

Scramble eggs and mix in a combination of veggies, such as spinach, tomato, and bell pepper

Serve with a whole grain English muffin

Lunch: Chickpea Salad

Mix chickpeas, cherry tomatoes, red onion, and cucumber in a bowl

Dress with a mixture of lemon juice, olive oil, and spices

Serve on a bed of mixed greens or in a whole grain pita

Dinner: Grilled Beef and Broccoli Stir Fry

Grill 4 ounces of sliced beef and stir fry with broccoli, garlic, and soy sauce

Serve over brown rice

Day 6:

Breakfast: Peanut Butter and Banana Smoothie

Blend almond milk, Greek yogurt, banana, and a tablespoon of peanut butter in a blender

Protein powder may be added, if desired.

Lunch: Tuna Salad

Mix canned tuna with chopped celery, red onion, and a small amount of mayonnaise

Serve on whole grain crackers or on a bed of mixed greens

Dinner: Baked Chicken with Roasted Vegetables

Preheat oven to 400°F

Bake 4 ounces of chicken breast in a baking dish

Roast a mixture of vegetables, such as carrots, Brussels sprouts, and red onion, in the oven

Serve with a side of brown rice.

Day 7:

Breakfast: Fruit and Yogurt Bowl

Layer Greek yogurt, mixed berries, sliced banana, and a handful of granola in a bowl

Repeat layers until ingredients are used up

Lunch: Turkey and Avocado Sandwich

Spread mashed avocado on a whole grain bread

Top with sliced turkey, tomato, and lettuce

Serve with a side of mixed greens

Dinner: Grilled Vegetable and Feta Salad

Grill a mixture of vegetables, such as zucchini, bell pepper, and eggplant

Serve on a bed of mixed greens with crumbled feta cheese and a dressing of olive oil and balsamic vinegar.

This meal plan emphasizes whole, unprocessed foods, lean protein, and plenty of vegetables. It provides a balance of carbohydrates, protein, and healthy fats to support weight loss and maintain energy levels throughout the day. Remember to drink plenty of water, stay active, and consult with a healthcare professional before starting any exercise program.

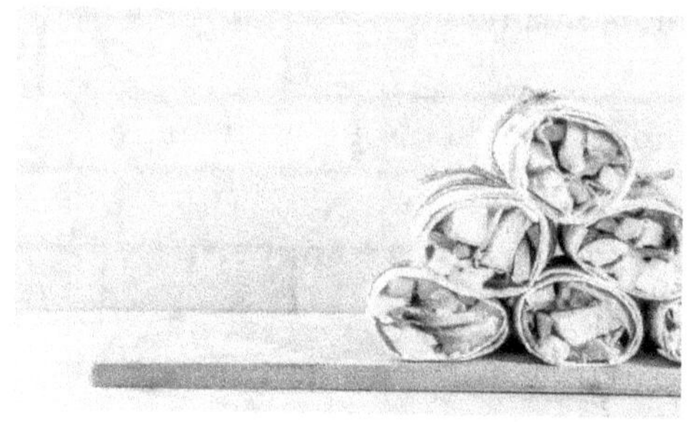

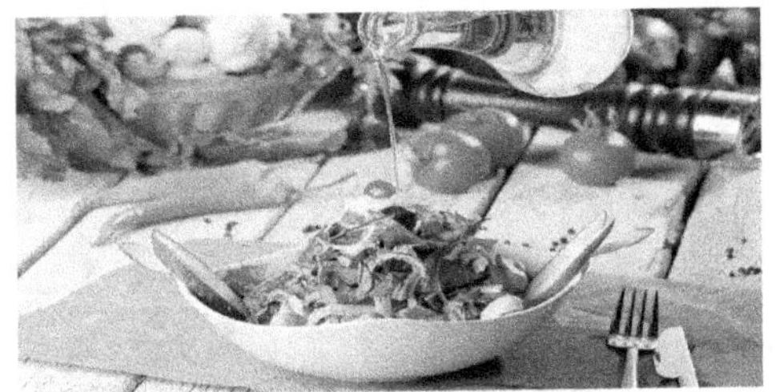

CHAPTER 4: PHYSICAL ACTIVITY AND EXERCISE

The Role of Physical Activity in Weight Loss

Physical activity is an important aspect of weight loss and overall health and wellness. Regular exercise, along with a balanced diet, can help individuals reach their weight loss goals and improve their overall health. Important roles that physical activity plays in weight loss include:

Burns Calories: One of the most straightforward ways physical activity helps with weight loss is by burning calories. When we engage in physical activity, our bodies burn calories, which helps to reduce the overall number of calories we consume. The result of this calorie shortfall can be weight loss.

Increases Metabolism: Physical activity can help increase our metabolism, which is the rate at which our bodies burn calories. This means that even when we are not actively exercising, our bodies are still burning calories at a higher rate, which can help with weight loss.

Builds Muscle Mass: Regular physical activity, especially strength training exercises, can help build muscle mass. Muscle tissue burns more calories than fat tissue, which means that increasing our muscle mass can help us burn more calories even when we are at rest.

Reduces Stress and Improves Mood: Physical activity has been shown to reduce stress and improve mood. When we feel stressed or down, it can be tempting to turn to junk food or overeat, which can lead to weight gain.

By engaging in regular physical activity, we can reduce stress, improve our mood, and reduce the likelihood of overeating and weight gain.

Increases Satiety: Physical activity can also help increase feelings of satiety, or fullness, which can reduce the likelihood of overeating and snacking between meals.

Promotes Long-Term Weight Management: Physical activity, combined with a balanced diet, can help promote long-term weight management. By regularly engaging in physical activity and making healthy food choices, we can maintain a healthy weight and reduce the likelihood of weight regain.

Improves Cardiovascular Health: In addition to helping with weight loss, physical activity also has numerous other health benefits, including improving cardiovascular health. Regular physical activity can help strengthen the heart and blood vessels, lower blood pressure, and reduce the risk of heart disease and stroke.

Increases Insulin Sensitivity: Physical activity can also help improve insulin sensitivity, which is crucial for managing blood sugar levels and reducing the risk of Type 2 diabetes. By improving insulin sensitivity, physical activity can help regulate blood sugar levels and promote overall health and wellness.

Boosts Confidence and Self-Esteem: Engaging in regular physical activity can also boost confidence and self-esteem. As we see the results of our hard work and become more physically fit, our self-esteem and confidence can improve, which can have a positive impact on our overall mental health and well-being.

In conclusion, physical exercises play important functions in weight loss. By burning calories, increasing metabolism, building muscle mass, reducing stress, and improving satiety, physical activity can help support and enhance the weight loss process. It is important to engage in regular physical activity as part of a comprehensive weight loss program that also includes a balanced diet and healthy lifestyle habits.

Types of Exercises and Their Benefits

There are many different types of exercises, each with their own set of benefits. They include:

Aerobic Exercise: This type of exercise involves continuous rhythmic movement of the large muscle groups, such as running, cycling, or swimming. Aerobic exercise is known to improve cardiovascular health, reduce the risk of chronic diseases such as heart disease and diabetes, improve lung function, and increase endurance.

Strength Training: Also known as resistance training or weightlifting, strength training involves using weights, resistance bands, or bodyweight exercises to build muscle strength and endurance. Benefits of strength training include improved muscle tone, increased bone density, improved posture, reduced risk of injury, and increased metabolism.

Flexibility Exercise: This type of exercise includes stretching and other movements that help improve range of motion and prevent injury. Benefits of flexibility exercises include improved posture, reduced risk of injury, increased joint mobility, and reduced stress.

High-Intensity Interval Training (HIIT): HIIT involves short, intense bursts of exercise followed by brief periods of rest. Benefits of HIIT include improved cardiovascular fitness, increased calorie burn, and improved endurance.

Yoga: This type of exercise combines physical poses, breathing techniques, and meditation to improve strength, flexibility, balance, and mental focus. Advantages of yoga include reduced stress, improved flexibility and balance, increased muscle strength, and improved overall fitness.

Pilates: Pilates involves a series of exercises designed to improve core strength, flexibility, and balance. Benefits of Pilates include improved posture, reduced risk of injury, increased muscle strength, and improved overall fitness.

However, some additional details on the benefits of different types of exercises:

Aerobic Exercise: Aerobic exercise helps improve cardiovascular health by strengthening the heart and lungs. This type of exercise can also help lower blood pressure, improve blood sugar control, and reduce the risk of stroke. Additionally, regular aerobic exercise can help improve mood, reduce anxiety and depression, and boost cognitive function.

Strength Training: Strength training is an effective way to increase muscle strength, endurance, and size. It can also help improve bone density, which is important for preventing osteoporosis. Additionally, strength training can help improve balance and reduce the risk of falls in older adults. It can also be helpful for people with certain medical conditions, such as arthritis or chronic back pain.

Flexibility Exercise: Flexibility exercises, such as stretching, can help improve joint mobility, reduce muscle tension, and improve posture. This type of exercise can also help reduce the risk of injury, particularly in athletes or people who engage in high-intensity exercise.

High-Intensity Interval Training (HIIT): HIIT can be a time-efficient way to improve cardiovascular fitness and burn calories. It has also been shown to improve insulin sensitivity and blood sugar control, making it a potential strategy for managing diabetes. Additionally, HIIT may be more effective than steady-state exercise for improving cardiovascular health in some populations, such as older adults or people with obesity.

Yoga: In addition to the physical benefits of yoga, such as improved flexibility and balance, this type of exercise has been shown to have mental health benefits as well. Yoga can help reduce stress, anxiety, and depression, and improve sleep quality. It may also improve cognitive function and help improve symptoms of conditions such as post-traumatic stress disorder (PTSD).

Pilates: Pilates can be helpful for people with chronic back pain, as it focuses on improving core strength and posture. This type of exercise can also help improve balance, flexibility, and muscle tone. Additionally, Pilates may be beneficial for people with conditions such as multiple sclerosis or Parkinson's disease, as it can help improve mobility and reduce symptoms.

Overall, engaging in regular exercise can have a multitude of benefits for both physical and mental health. It is important to choose a variety of exercises that work different muscle groups and incorporate both aerobic and strength training for optimal health benefits.

Creating an effective exercise plan

Here is a simple and effective exercise plan for weight loss:

Brisk walking: Walking is a low-impact exercise that is easy to incorporate into your daily routine. Start with a 10-minute walk, gradually increasing the time to 30 minutes or more. Aim to walk at a brisk pace to increase your heart rate and burn more calories.

Interval training: Interval training involves alternating between high-intensity exercise and rest periods. You can try sprinting for 30 seconds and then walking for 60 seconds, or doing jumping jacks for 30 seconds and then resting for 30 seconds. Repeat for 10-20 minutes.

Strength training: Strength training helps build muscle, which burns more calories even at rest.

Start with bodyweight exercises like squats, lunges, and push-ups, and gradually increase the weight or resistance as you get stronger.

Yoga: Yoga can help improve flexibility, balance, and core strength, all of which can aid in weight loss. Try a beginner's yoga class or follow a video tutorial at home.

Cardiovascular exercise: Cardiovascular exercise, such as running, cycling, or swimming, can help burn calories and improve your cardiovascular health. Start with 10-15 minutes of moderate intensity exercise and gradually increase the time and intensity over time.

HIIT: High-Intensity Interval Training (HIIT) is a form of cardio exercise that alternates between short bursts of intense activity and rest periods. HIIT can help you burn calories quickly and efficiently, even in a short amount of time.

Dance workouts: Dancing is a fun and effective way to burn calories and improve your cardiovascular health.

You can join a dance class or follow a dance workout video at home.

Circuit training: Circuit training involves completing a series of exercises one after the other with little or no rest in between. By doing so, you'll be able to lose weight and increase your general level of fitness. You can do a circuit of bodyweight exercises or use weights or resistance bands.

Consistency is key when it comes to weight loss. Aim to exercise at least 30 minutes a day, five days a week. You can also mix and match different exercises to keep your routine interesting and challenging.

Remember, the most important thing is to find an exercise routine that you enjoy and that you can stick with. Don't be afraid to try new things and mix up your workouts to keep things interesting.

And always consult with a healthcare professional before starting a new exercise routine, especially if you have any underlying health conditions.

Incorporating physical activity into a busy lifestyle

Adding exercises to a busy lifestyle for weight loss can be challenging, but here are some helpful tips:

Set achievable goals: Start with small, achievable goals that fit into your schedule. For example, aim to exercise for 10-15 minutes a day, three times a week.

Schedule your workouts: Treat your workouts like important appointments and schedule them in your calendar. Make them a priority, and stick to your schedule as much as possible.

Find opportunities to be active: Look for ways to incorporate physical activity into your daily routine, such as taking the stairs instead of the elevator or going for a walk during your lunch break.

Try high-intensity interval training (HIIT): HIIT workouts can be done in a short amount of time and are very effective for weight loss. They involve short bursts of intense exercise followed by periods of rest.

Use technology: There are many apps and online resources available that offer quick and effective workouts that can be done at home or on-the-go.

Be consistent: Consistency is key when it comes to weight loss. Make exercise a habit, and stick to your routine as much as possible.

Some additional tips to help you add exercises to a busy lifestyle for weight loss:

Wake up earlier: If your schedule is packed during the day, consider waking up earlier to fit in a workout. Even just 30 minutes of exercise in the morning can help jumpstart your metabolism and give you more energy throughout the day.

Make it a family affair: If you have children or a partner, get them involved in your exercise routine. Plan activities like hiking, biking, or playing sports together, or take turns watching the kids while the other person works out.

Join a gym or fitness class: If you have trouble staying motivated on your own, consider joining a gym or fitness class. This can help keep you accountable and provide structure to your workouts.

Mix it up: Doing the same workout routine over and over can get boring and make it harder to stick to your exercise goals. Try different types of exercises to keep things interesting and challenging, such as yoga, weightlifting, or swimming.

Use your lunch break: If you work outside of the home, use your lunch break to squeeze in a quick workout. Go for a walk or jog, or do some strength training exercises in a nearby park.

Stay active throughout the day: In addition to scheduled workouts, find ways to stay active throughout the day. Take breaks to stretch and move around if you work at a desk, or take the stairs instead of the elevator. Every little bit of activity adds up!

Remember, the most important thing is to find a routine that works for you and that you can stick to. With consistency and dedication, you can add exercise to your busy lifestyle and achieve your weight loss goals.

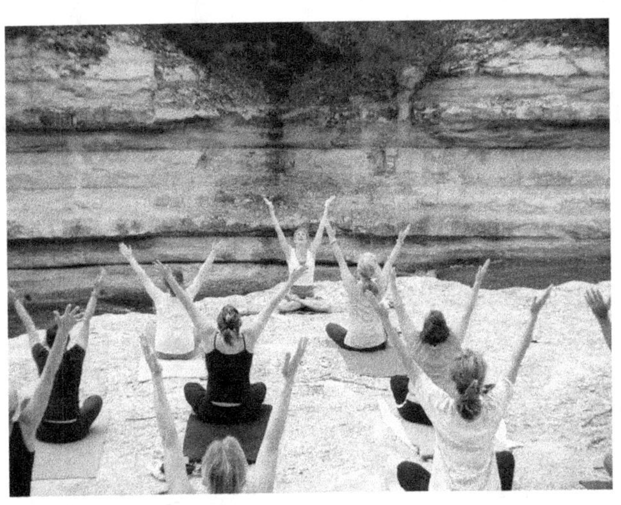

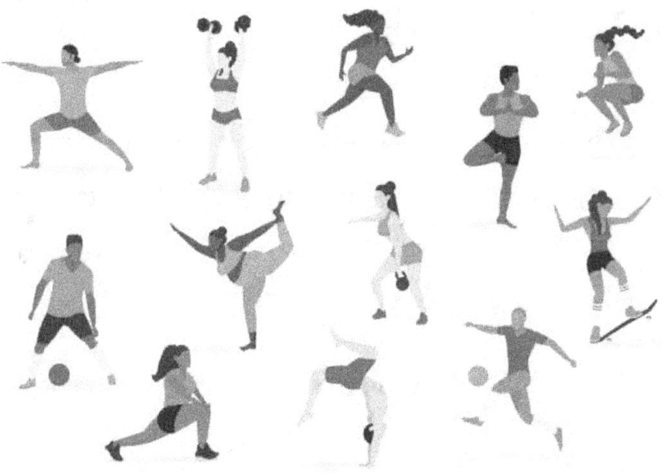

CHAPTER 5: IMPLEMENTING A SUSTAINABLE WEIGHT LOSS PLAN

Understanding the Difference between a Quick Fix and Sustainable Weight Loss

The desire to lose weight quickly is a common one, but it's important to be aware of the distinction between weight loss that is lasting and a rapid fix.

Some key considerations to keep in mind include:

Sustainable changes: A rapid fix for weight loss, such as a crash diet or extreme workout regimen, may result in quick weight loss, but it is unlikely to be sustainable over the long-term. Instead, focus on making gradual, sustainable changes to your diet and exercise habits that you can maintain for the rest of your life.

This could include adding more whole foods to your diet, increasing your daily physical activity, and finding enjoyable forms of exercise that you can stick to.

Slow and steady progress: It's important to be patient when it comes to weight loss. Losing weight too quickly can be harmful to your health and may lead to rebound weight gain. Aim for a slow and steady rate of weight loss, such as 1-2 pounds per week, which is a safe and sustainable rate of progress.

Lifestyle changes: Focus on making lifestyle changes that you can sustain over the long term, rather than quick fixes that may only offer temporary results. This includes adopting healthy habits such as drinking enough water, getting enough sleep, and managing stress.

Support system: Build a support system that can help you stay accountable and motivated on your weight loss journey. This could include friends, family, or a professional coach or counselor.

Mindset shift: Adopt a growth mindset that allows for learning and improvement over time, rather than a fixed mindset that sees weight loss as an all-or-nothing proposition. Celebrate small victories along the way and focus on progress rather than perfection.

Tracking progress: Keeping track of your progress can be helpful in maintaining motivation and staying on track towards your weight loss goals. This can be done by tracking your food intake, exercise, and weight, as well as taking measurements of your body.

Variety: Incorporate variety into your diet and exercise routine to keep things interesting and prevent boredom or burnout. This could include trying new healthy recipes, exploring different forms of exercise, or mixing up your workout routine.

Self-care: It's important to take care of yourself both physically and mentally while on your weight loss journey. This could include practicing stress-reducing techniques, prioritizing self-care activities, and seeking support if you are struggling with body image issues or disordered eating.

Long-term focus: Remember that lasting weight loss is a marathon, not a sprint. It's important to maintain a long-term focus and continue making healthy choices even after you have reached your goal weight. This will help you maintain your weight loss and improve your overall health in the long run.

Patience and kindness: Finally, be patient and kind to yourself. Weight loss can be a challenging journey, but it's important to approach it with a positive and compassionate mindset. Be proud of your progress and celebrate the small victories along the way, even if they are not directly related to weight loss.

In conclusion, lasting weight loss requires a holistic approach that involves making sustainable lifestyle changes, building a support system, and taking care of yourself both physically and mentally. By adopting a growth mindset, focusing on slow and steady progress, and maintaining a long-term focus, you can achieve your weight loss goals in a healthy and sustainable way.

Modifying one's food habits and degree of exercise gradually

Modifying dietary practices and exercise levels gradually can be a sustainable way to improve overall health and well-being.

The following advice will help you implement these changes:

Set realistic goals: When it comes to eating habits and physical activity, it's important to set achievable goals. Build up progressively over time by beginning small. For example, aim to walk for 10 minutes a day, and then gradually increase to 30 minutes a day.

Keep a food journal: Keeping track of what you eat can help you identify areas for improvement. Write down everything you eat and drink for a week, and then review your journal to see where you can make changes.

Focus on whole foods: Try to eat more whole foods, such as fruits, vegetables, whole grains, lean protein, and healthy fats. These foods provide essential nutrients and can help you feel fuller for longer.

Reduce portion sizes: Eating smaller portions can help you reduce your overall calorie intake. Use a smaller plate, and take your time when eating to give your brain time to register that you're full.

Make healthy swaps: Instead of reaching for a candy bar, choose a piece of fruit. Drink water or unsweetened tea instead of sugar-laden beverages.

Incorporate physical activity into your day: Take the stairs instead of the elevator, walk instead of drive for short distances, or do some light exercises during commercial breaks while watching TV.

Discover activities you like: It's not necessary for exercise to be a hassle. Make some enjoyable activity a regular part of your schedule, whether it be swimming, hiking, or dancing.

Get support: Making changes to your eating habits and physical activity can be challenging, but having support can make a big difference. Enlist the help of a friend or family member, or consider working with a personal trainer or nutritionist.

Remember, the key to making gradual changes is to be patient and persistent. Over time, small changes can lead to big improvements in your health and well-being.

Staying on track and avoiding common obstacles

Below are some ways to stay on track and avoid common obstacles in weight loss:

Set realistic goals: Avoid setting unattainable or overly ambitious goals. Instead, set smaller, achievable goals that can be built upon over time.

Plan meals and snacks: Create a meal plan for the week that includes a variety of healthy foods. Plan ahead for snacks to avoid reaching for unhealthy options when hunger strikes.

Stay active: Incorporate regular exercise into your routine. This can be as simple as going for a daily walk or taking up a new activity.

Find support: Seek out a friend or family member to be your accountability partner or join a support group to stay motivated.

Monitor progress: Keep track of your weight loss progress and celebrate milestones. This will help keep you motivated and on track.

Avoid temptations: Remove unhealthy foods from your home and avoid situations where you may be tempted to overeat or indulge in unhealthy habits.

Get enough sleep: Lack of sleep can disrupt hormone levels and metabolism, leading to weight gain. Attempt to get 7-8 hours of sleep each night.

Don't give up: Weight loss is a journey that requires time and effort. Don't get discouraged if progress is slow or if there are setbacks along the way. To achieve your goals, remain dedicated and focused.

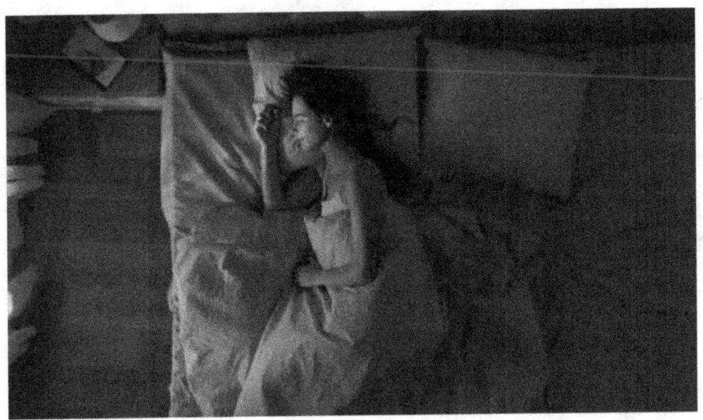

CHAPTER 6: MAINTAINING A HEALTHY WEIGHT

The Importance of maintaining weight loss

Continuing to lose weight can have significant benefits for both physical and mental health.

Some advantages of weight loss are:

Improved physical health: Losing weight can help reduce the risk of developing chronic diseases such as type 2 diabetes, heart disease, and stroke. It can also improve overall physical function and mobility, making it easier to perform daily activities and reducing the risk of injuries.

Increased energy: Losing weight can increase energy levels, making it easier to engage in physical activity and improve overall quality of life.

Boosted confidence: Achieving weight loss goals can boost confidence and self-esteem, improving overall mental health and wellbeing.

Better sleep: Losing weight can help reduce snoring and sleep apneas, leading to better sleep quality and more restful nights.

Long-term health benefits: Maintaining a healthy weight over time can lead to a longer, healthier life with fewer health complications.

However, it's essential to approach weight loss in a healthy, sustainable way, focusing on balanced nutrition and regular exercise, rather than quick fixes or fad diets.

Strategies for Avoiding Weight Regain

Some strategies to avoid weight regain:

Maintain a healthy diet: Focus on a balanced diet that includes whole foods, lean proteins, healthy fats, and complex carbohydrates. Avoid processed and high-calorie foods.

Increase physical activity: Exercise is an essential factor in weight loss and maintenance. Regular exercises help to burn calories and maintain muscle mass.

Stay hydrated: Drinking water can help in maintaining a healthy weight by boosting metabolism and reducing appetite.

Regularly monitor your weight: Keeping track of your weight will help you to identify early signs of weight gain and make necessary changes in your diet and exercise routine.

Set realistic goals: Set new achievable goals for weight loss and make a plan for how to maintain them.

Avoid emotional eating: Emotional eating is a common reason for weight gain. Instead of resorting to food for comfort, develop healthy coping strategies.

Get enough sleep: Sleep deprivation can lead to weight gain. Consistently aim for seven to eight hours of sleep each night.

Keep yourself motivated: Staying motivated is key to avoiding weight regain. Join support groups, work with a weight loss coach or therapist to help you stay motivated.

Avoid alcohol: Drinking alcohol can lead to overeating and weight gain. Consider reducing or quitting drinking entirely.

Managing your stress is important; it will prevent you from gaining weight. **Few ways to manage stress are meditation, yoga, or deep breathing exercises.**

Plan your meals ahead of time: Meal planning can help you avoid impulsive food choices, overeating, and snacking on unhealthy foods.

Practice mindful eating: Pay attention to your hunger cues, chew your food slowly, and savor each bite. This can help you to eat less and feel more satisfied.

Take breaks from sitting: Sitting for long periods of time can lead to weight gain. Take short breaks throughout the day to stand up, stretch, and move your body.

Avoid skipping meals because doing so can cause you to overeat later in the day. Make sure to eat regular meals and snacks throughout the day.

Celebrate your progress: Celebrate your progress and success along the way. This can help you to stay motivated and continue with your healthy habits.

In summary, maintaining a healthy weight requires consistent effort, but following these strategies can help you avoid weight regain and stay on track with your health and fitness goals. Remember to be patient, stay motivated, and celebrate your success along the way.

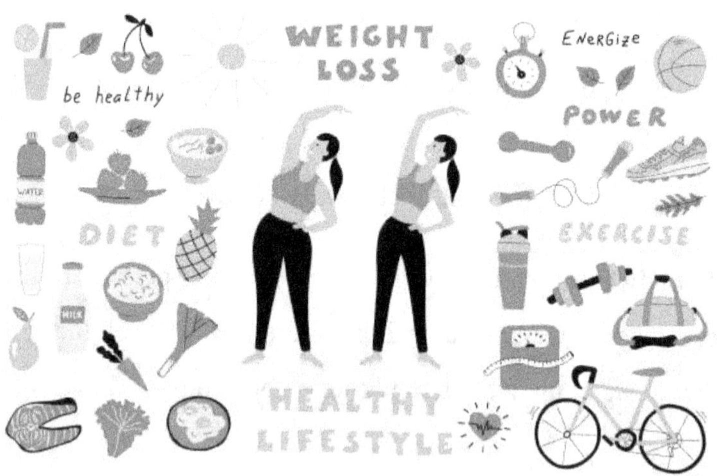

Incorporating Healthy Habits into a Long-Term Lifestyle

Set realistic and achievable goals: Setting achievable goals is crucial when trying to make healthful practices a permanent part of one's lifestyle. Start with small goals such as walking for 20 minutes every day or adding more vegetables to your meals. Gradually increase your goals as you start to see progress.

Find an exercise routine you enjoy: Incorporating exercise into your lifestyle is essential for losing weight and maintaining good health. Whether it's dance, yoga, or jogging, choose a fitness program that you like. This will help you stick to it and make it a habit.

Meal prep: Plan your meals in advance and make sure they are packed with nutrient-dense foods. Meal prepping ensures that you always have healthy options available and saves time and money.

Practice mindfulness: Mindfulness can help you become more aware of your eating habits and make conscious decisions about what you put into your body. This includes paying attention to hunger and fullness cues and avoiding mindless snacking.

Stay accountable: Having a support system and holding yourself accountable can help you stay motivated and on track. Consider joining a weight loss group or finding a workout partner to keep you accountable.

Don't deprive yourself: It's important to allow yourself treats in moderation. Completely cutting out foods you love can lead to cravings and binge eating. Instead, indulge in moderation and savor every bite.

Keep track of progress: Tracking your progress, whether it's through a journal or an app, can help you see how far you've come and motivate you to keep going. Celebrate small victories and use setbacks as an opportunity to learn and grow.

Remember, losing weight and making healthful practices a permanent part of your lifestyle is a journey, not a destination. Be patient and kind to yourself, and embrace the process.

Get enough sleep: Sleep is essential for overall health and weight loss. Your hormones can be upset and your hunger increased by lack of sleep, which can make you eat more than you should. Spend seven to eight hours each night getting a good night's sleep.

Practice stress-reducing activities: Stress can lead to emotional eating and weight gain. Use relaxation techniques to reduce your stress levels, such as yoga, meditation, or deep breathing. You can decompress and lessen your stress by engaging in these activities.

Make it a lifestyle: The key to making healthful practices a permanent part of your lifestyle is to make them a habit. Incorporate healthy eating and exercise into your daily routine, and make it a priority. Eventually, these habits will become second nature, and you won't even have to think about them.

CONCLUSION

Weight loss and its maintenance are essential components of maintaining a healthy lifestyle. It involves the process of reducing one's body weight, maintaining the achieved weight and avoiding weight gain. It has become a significant concern in today's society, where the prevalence of obesity and overweight is increasing worldwide.

Numerous strategies have been recommended for weight loss, including healthy eating habits, regular physical exercise, and behavior modification techniques.

Healthy eating habits such as reducing calorie intake and choosing foods with a low glycemic index have proven to be effective in achieving weight loss.

Physical activity also plays a crucial role in weight loss as it burns calories and enhances metabolism. Behavior modification techniques such as self-monitoring, goal-setting, and social support have also been shown to be effective in maintaining a healthy weight.

Weight maintenance, on the other hand, involves sustaining the lost weight over time.

This is often challenging as the body is prone to regain weight due to various factors such as genetics, metabolism, and lifestyle changes.

One of the key strategies for weight maintenance is adopting healthy eating and physical activity habits that promote energy balance. These include eating a balanced diet that provides adequate nutrition and physical exercise that is enjoyable and sustainable.

Another essential aspect of weight maintenance is developing a positive mindset towards weight loss and maintenance. This involves having realistic goals and expectations, practicing self-compassion, and avoiding negative self-talk. It is also crucial to have a supportive social network that provides encouragement and accountability.

It is important to note that weight loss and maintenance are not just about appearance, but also about overall health and well-being. Obesity and overweight have been linked to various health conditions, including diabetes, heart disease, and some cancers. Maintaining a healthy weight helps to reduce the risk of these conditions and promotes overall health.

In conclusion, weight loss and maintenance are vital for a healthy lifestyle. The process involves healthy eating habits; physical activity, behavior modification techniques, and positive mindset, all of which promote weight loss and help sustain it over time.

Adopting and maintaining these practices can lead to better health outcomes and overall well-being.

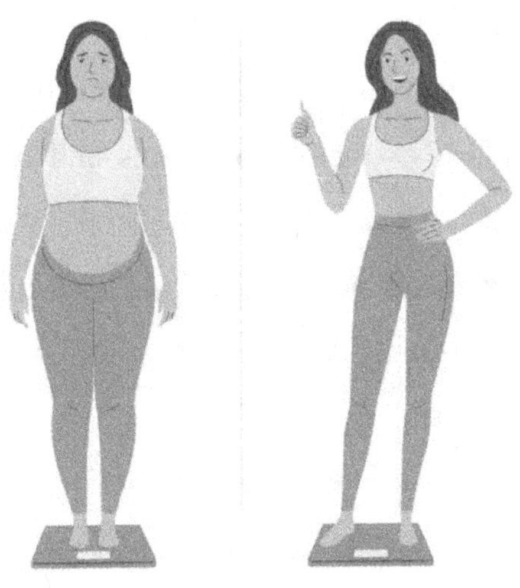

SUMMARY OF KEY TAKEAWAYS

Here are some of the main conclusions on weight loss:

- You must consume less calories than you burn each day in order to lose weight. It is refer to as a calorie deficit.

- For weight loss to work, consistency is essential. It's important to maintain a healthy diet and exercise routine over an extended period of time to achieve sustainable weight loss.

- Crash diets or extreme calorie restriction are not effective or sustainable ways to lose weight. They may result in short-term weight loss, but they can also lead to health problems and rebound weight gain.

- A balanced and varied diet that includes whole, nutrient-dense foods is essential for weight loss and overall health.

- Physical activity is important for weight loss, but it's not necessary to engage in extreme or high-intensity exercise. Consistent, moderate-intensity exercise can be effective for weight loss.

- Getting enough sleep is important for weight loss. It may be more difficult to lose weight if hormones that control metabolism and appetite are disrupted by sleep deprivation.

- Fad diets, such as those that eliminate entire food groups or rely on supplements, are not effective or sustainable for weight loss.

- Weight loss medications or surgery may be options for some individuals, but they should only be considered after other methods of weight loss have been tried and have not been successful.

- Weight loss can have significant health benefits, including reducing the risk of chronic diseases such as diabetes and heart disease.

- Drinking water can help you lose weight. Studies have shown that drinking water before meals can help reduce calories intake and boost weight loss.

- A support system can help with weight loss. Having support a support system, whether friends, family or weight loss group, can provide accountability and encouragement.

- Drinking alcohol can hinder weight loss. Alcoholic drinks are often high in calories and can lower inhibitions, leading to overeating and poor food choices.

In conclusion, achieving and maintaining a healthy weight is a journey that requires commitment, dedication, and hard work. It is not a one-time event, but a lifestyle change that must be adopted for a lifetime.

This book has provided you with valuable insights, practical tips, and effective strategies that can help you lose weight and keep it off for good.

Remember that losing weight is not just about looking good or fitting into your favorite clothes; it's about improving your overall health and wellbeing. By shedding those extra pounds, you can reduce your risk of chronic diseases, boost your energy levels, and enjoy a better quality of life.

The key to success is to set realistic goals, stay motivated, and be consistent with your efforts. It's okay to have setbacks and slip-ups, but what's important is that you keep pushing forward and never give up.

With the right mindset, support, and resources, you can achieve your weight loss goals and become the best version of yourself.

Thank you for choosing this book as your guide on this journey. I wish you all the best in your weight loss endeavors and a happier, healthier life ahead.